Ultimat
Copycat Cookbook
2021

Discover unique dishes and recipes from famous restaurants. Take inspiration from Olive Garden, Cheesecake Factory and Cracker Barrel to impress your friends at dinner.

Jaqueline Weber

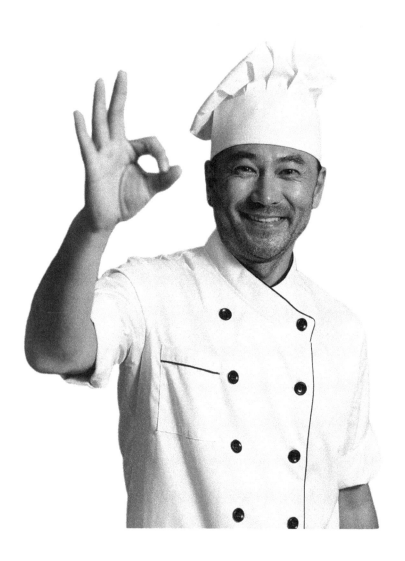

TABLE OF CONTENTS

INTRODUCTION

Meals in the restaurant can contain several unhealthy ingredients. There is also much more than what you lack when you feed on a take-outs.

These are some explanations of why you should consider having your cooking dinner tonight!

A Nutrient-Dense Plate

If prepared food arrives from outside the home, you typically have limited knowledge about salt, sugar, and processed oils. For a fact, we also apply more to our meal when it is served to the table. You will say how much salt, sugar, and oil are being used to prepare meals at home.

Increased Fruit and Vegetable Intake

The typical western diet loses both the weight and durability of plant foods we need to preserve. Many People eat only two fresh fruit and vegetables a day, while at least five portions are required. Tons of premade food, like restaurant food goods, restrict fruit and vegetable parts.

By supplying you with the convenience of cooking at home, you have complete control over your food. The message to note is that your attention will continue with the intake of more fruit and vegetables. Attach them to your cooking, snack them, or exchange them with your relatives on their way. Then take steps towards organic alternatives. It is always better to eat entire fruits and vegetables, whether or not organic, than processed foods.

Save Money and Use What You Have

Just because you haven't visited your local health food or food store this week doesn't mean you get stuck with taking in. Open your cupboard and fridge and see what you can make for a meal. It can be as easy as gluten-free rice, roasted tomatoes, carrots, frozen vegetables, and lemon juice. This simple meal is packed with fiber, protein, vitamins, and minerals. Best of all, in less than 30 minutes, it is delicious and can be prepared. You can save up your money in the long run and allows you sufficient food to share with or break the next day.

Sensible Snacking

Bringing premade snacks saves time, but everything goes back to what's in these products still. Don't worry, you can still have your guilty pleasures, but there is a way to make them more nutritious and often taste better. Swap your chips and dip the chopped vegetables into hummus. Create your snacks with bagged potato chips or carrots. Take a bowl and make your popcorn on top of your stove or in the popcorn machine. You can manage the amount of salt, sugar, and oil added.

Share Your Delicious Health

Once you make your recipes, you are so proud of your achievements. Furthermore, the food tastes amazing. Don't confuse me now–some of your inventive recipes won't taste the same thing, but friends and family will love your cuisine with constant practice and experimentation. You will see them enjoy the best nutritious food because of you and your faith in spreading health and love.

It Gives You a Chance to Reconnect

Having that chance to cook together helps you reconnect with your partner and your loved ones. Cooking also has other benefits. The American Psychological Association says that working together with new things—like learning a new recipe—can help maintain a relationship.

It's Proven to Be Healthier

Many researchers say that those who eat more often than not have a healthier diet overall. Such studies also show that in restaurants, menus, salt, saturated fat, total fat, and average calories are typically higher than in-house diets.

You have complete control over your food, whether you put fresh products together or shipped them straight to your door using a company like Plated. It can make a difference in your overall health.

It's Easier to Watch Your Calories

The average fast-food order is between 1,100 and 1,200 calories in total—nearly all the highly recommended daily calorie intake is 1,600 to 2,400 calories by a woman and almost two thirds (2,000 to 3,000 calories) a man daily. So, think again if you felt the independent restaurants so smaller chains would do well. Such products suck up an average of 1.327 calories per meal of additional calories.

Creating your food ensures you can guarantee that the portion sizes and calories are where you want them. Recipes also come with nutritional information and tips for sizing, which ease this.

It's a Time Saver

Part of shopping is to wait for food to come or travel to get it. It may take much more time, depending on where you live, what time you order, and whether or not the delivery person is good at directions!

It doesn't have to take much time to cook at home if you don't want it. You remove the need to search for ingredients or foodstuffs by using a service like Plated. Everything you need is at your house, in the exact amount that you use.

It's Personalized

Cooking at home gives you the chance to enjoy the food you want, how you like it. For starters, with Plated, if you want your meat more well-done or less sweet, the formula includes suggested changes.

Enjoying the Process

Once you come back home from a busy day, there is little more enjoyable than disconnecting from work emails, voicemails, unfinished assignments, or homework. Cooking at home presents you with a break from your routine and space for imagination. Rather than listen to noisy messages, you should put on the radio, collect spices, and reflect on the sizzle's odors on the stove or roast vegetables. It may stun you on how much you might like it when you make a daily habit of preparing food.

If your breakfast is great, lunch soup, or fresh tomato sauce for dinner, home cooking is a worthy investment. In return for your time and energy in preparation, you will benefit richly—from cost savings to fun with friends.

And the more you enjoy cooking in the kitchen, the more you get to make fantastic food!

BREAKFAST AND BRUNCH RECIPES

Asiago Cheese Bread

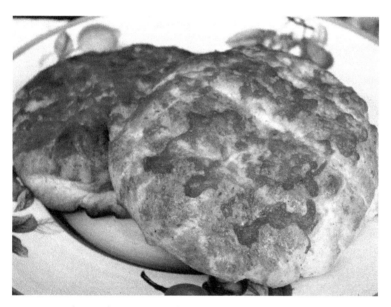

Preparation Time: 45 minutes

Cooking Time: 35 minutes

Servings: 20

Ingredients

- 1 ½ cups shredded Asiago cheese divided
- 3 ¼ cups all-purpose flour

- 1 beaten egg, large
- 1 ¼ cups milk
- 1 teaspoon granulated sugar
- ¼ teaspoon black pepper
- 1 pack Red Star Platinum Superior Baking Yeast
- 2 tablespoons butter
- 1 ½ teaspoons salt

Directions

1. Combine 1 ½ cups of flour together with sugar, yeast, pepper and salt in the bowl of a stand mixer. Pour in milk in a microwave safe bowl. Melt butter over moderate heat. Transfer milk mixture into the flour mixture & mix on low speed using the paddle attachment. Stir in 1 ¼ cups of shredded cheese; mix until just combined.

2. Slowly add in 1 ¾ cups of flour; knead until you get soft dough like consistency. Knead using stand mixer with the dough hook for 5 minutes.

3. Spray a bowl lightly with the cooking spray. Add the dough to the bowl and then turn the dough. Cover the bowl & let the dough to rise for an hour or two, until almost double, in a warm place.

4. Once done, punch the dough down & form it into two loaves. Place the loaves on a large-sized baking sheet, lightly coated with the cooking spray. Cover the loaves & let rise again for 35 to 40 minutes, until doubled.

5. Preheat your oven to 375 F in advance.

6. Using a serrated knife; make a few cuts in the top of loaves. Egg washes the tops of the loaves then sprinkle the leftover cheese. Bake in the preheated oven until lightly browned, for 30 to 35 minutes.

Nutrition: 840 calories 54g total fats 34g protein

Roadhouse Mashed Potatoes

Preparation Time: 20 minutes

Cooking Time: 30 minutes

Servings: 6

Ingredients

- ¼ cup Parmesan cheese, grated
- 1 whole garlic bulb
- ¼ cup sour cream
- 4 medium potatoes, peeled & quartered
- ¼ cup each of softened butter & 2% milk
- 1 teaspoon plus 1 tablespoon olive oil
- ¼ teaspoon pepper
- 1 medium white onion, chopped
- ½ teaspoon salt

Directions

1. Preheat oven at 425 degrees. Cut off the papery outer skin from garlic bulb; ensure that you don't separate the cloves or peel them. Remove the top from the garlic bulb, exposing individual cloves. Brush cut cloves with approximately 1 teaspoon of oil then, wrap in foil. Bake for 33 minutes

2. Meanwhile, cook the leftover oil over low heat. Once done; add & cook the chopped onion for 15 to 20 minutes, until golden brown, stirring every now and

then. Transfer to a food processor. Process on high until blended well; set aside.

3. Situate potatoes in a big saucepan and cover them with water. Bring to a boil. Once done; decrease the heat; cook for 15 to 20 minutes, until tender, uncovered. Drain; return to the pan. Squeeze the softened garlic over the potatoes; add butter, cheese, sour cream, milk, onion, pepper and salt. Beat until mashed. Serve and enjoy

Nutrition: 220 calories 15g total fats 3g protein

Sweet Potatoes with Marshmallows and Caramel Sauce

Preparation Time: 40 minutes

Cooking Time: 30 minutes

Servings: 10

Ingredients

- ½ cup corn syrup
- 6 medium sweet potatoes
- ½ teaspoon ground cinnamon
- ¼ cup whole milk
- 2 tablespoons butter
- ½ cup brown sugar, packed
- Marshmallows on top
- ½ to 1 teaspoon salt

Directions

1. Put sweet potatoes in a Dutch oven; add water and ensure that the sweet potatoes are nicely covered. Bring to a boil. Once done; decrease the heat; cover & let simmer for 20 minutes.
2. Drain & transfer to a lightly greased 13x9" baking dish. Bake for 12 to 15 minutes, at 325 F, uncovered.
3. In the meantime, combine the leftover ingredients (except the marshmallows) together in a small saucepan. Bring to a boil; pour the mixture on top of

the sweet potatoes. Bake until glazed, for 10 to15 more minutes, basting frequently. Just before serving; throw some marshmallows on top. Enjoy.

Nutrition: 180 calories 12g total fats 4g protein

Sautéed Mushrooms

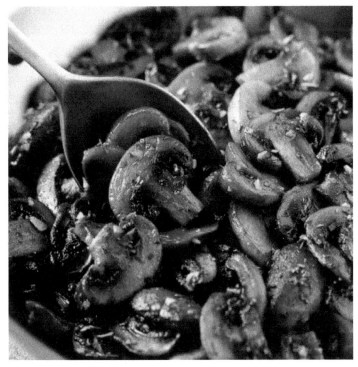

Preparation Time: 20 minutes

Cooking Time: 20 minutes

Servings: 6

Ingredients

- 1 teaspoon garlic, chopped
- 1 tablespoon butter
- 1 cup cleaned Portobello mushrooms, sliced
- 1 tablespoon thyme leaves, chopped
- 1/8 cup vegetable oil
- Freshly ground black pepper & salt to taste

Directions

1. Warm up the oil over high heat in a large skillet until hot & smoky. Add the garlic; cook until turn fragrant, toss it constantly and ensure that the garlic doesn't burn. Add the mushrooms; toss until mushrooms are caramelized and turn golden brown. Remove from the heat. Add butter and thyme; season with pepper and salt, to taste. Serve immediately & enjoy.

Nutrition: 191 calories 13g total fats 5g protein

Ham and Cheese Empanadas

Preparation Time: 5 minutes

Cooking Time: 15 minutes

Serving: 6

Ingredients

- 12 cooked ham feta
- 400 g mozzarella cheese
- 12 empanada tapas
- Dried oregano
- Ground chili pepper
- 1 beaten egg

Directions:

2. Cut the mozzarella cheese into 12 bars of approximately 30-35 g each. Pass the bars with oregano and floor chili pepper and area them in the center of each ham feta. Wrap the cheese with the ham, forming a bundle and reserve.

3. Stretch the dough of the empanadas a touch so that they're oval and location the applications of cheese and ham in the middle of each one in all them.

4. Close the middle and location a finger inside to push the ham even as persevering with to close the sides. This is so that the ham does not complicate your existence at the time of creating the repulse. Make the traditional replunge and forestalls placed them in an

appropriate greased baking sheet with oil. Paint the pies ham and cheese with crushed egg if desired and takes a warm oven till their golden brown.

5. If you want to fry ham and cheese empanadas, consider that the oil must be at 150-160 ° C, because if it had been hotter, they would be cooked on the outside and inside the cheese could no longer melt. Fry them for about 3 minutes. Remove the patties fried ham and cheese with a slotted spoon and depart them on paper towels to cast off extra oil.

Nutrition: 188 calories 16g total fats 11g protein

Roadhouse Green Beans

Preparation Time: 10 minutes

Cooking Time: 20 minutes

Servings: 8

Ingredients

- 2 cans green beans (16 ounce), drained
- 1 tablespoon sugar
- 4 ounces bacon, diced (raw) or 4 ounces ham (cooked)
- 2 cups water
- 4 ounces onions, diced
- ½ teaspoon pepper

Directions

1. Thoroughly drain green beans using a colander; set aside. Combine pepper with sugar & water until incorporated well; set aside. Preheat your cooking pan over medium high heat.

2. Dice the cooked ham into equal size pieces using a cutting board and a knife. Place the diced onions and ham into the preheated cooking pan. Continue to stir the onions and ham using the large spoon until the onions are tender and the ham is lightly brown.

3. Once done; add the beans and liquid mixture. Using the rubber spatula; give the mixture a good stir until incorporated well. Let the mixture to boil then lower the

heat to simmer. Serve the beans as soon as you are ready and enjoy.

Nutrition: 221 calories 16g total fats 4g protein

PASTA RECIPES

Linguine Carbonara

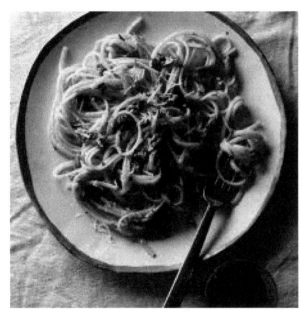

Preparation Time: 10 minutes

Cooking Time: 15 minutes

Servings: 4

Ingredients:

- 12 oz. linguine
- 6 oz. sliced bacon (cut into 1-inch pieces)
- 3 large egg yolks
- 1/2 c. freshly grated Parmesan

- 1/4 tsp. salt
- 1/4 tsp. pepper
- 1/2 c. chopped parsley

Directions:

1. Linguine to eat. Boil water for cooking then drains pasta.
2. Cook the bacon with medium-sized skillet. Transfer to a towel-lined sheet of paper.
3. Whisk egg yolks together, freshly grated Parmesan, and salt and pepper in a large bowl.
4. Little by little whisk warm cooking water in 1/4 cup reserved.
5. Add hot pasta and stir to coat, adding more water if the pasta appears dry.
6. Fold in the bacon and the chopped parsley. If needed, serve with lots of chopped pepper and extra Parmesan.

Nutrition: 256 Calories 14g Fat 10g Protein

Grilled Ratatouille Linguine

Preparation Time: 5 minutes

Cooking Time: 10 minutes

Servings: 4

Ingredients:

- 12 oz. linguine
- 2 small zucchinis, halved lengthwise
- 1 small eggplant, sliced lengthwise
- 1 red pepper, halved
- 1 yellow pepper, halved
- 1 red onion, cut into rounds
- 2 tbsp. olive oil
- Salt
- Pepper
- Grated Parmesan and chopped basil, if desired

Directions:

1. Heat to medium-high barbecue. Cook the linguine per directions for each kit.
2. Meanwhile, brush the zucchini, the eggplant, the peppers and the red oil onion and season each salt and pepper with 1/2 teaspoon.
3. Grill for 8 minutes both sides. Switch to a board to cut and cut into pieces.
4. Toss linguine with grilled vegetables and drizzle with as much oil as you wish.

5. Cover with finely diced basil and Parmesan.

Nutrition: 246 Calories 18g Fat 9g Protein

Shrimp and Zucchini Scampi

Preparation Time: 5 minutes

Cooking Time: 10 minutes

Servings: 6

Ingredients:

- 1 1/2 lb. shelled, deveined shrimp
- 2 tbsp. oil
- 2 medium zucchinis, sliced
- 4 cloves garlic, chopped
- 4 tbsp. butter
- 3/4 c. white wine
- 1/8 tsp. salt
- 1 lb. linguine, cooked
- 1/4 c. pasta cooking water
- 2 tsp. lemon peel, grated
- Chopped parsley, for serving

Directions:

1. Cook the shrimp in oil for 3 minutes or until ready to eat, turning once.
2. Place the shrimp on the tray.
3. Attach the zucchini, garlic and butter to skillet.
4. Cook for 3 mins. Add white wine and salt; cook, stirring and scraping for 2 minutes.
5. Sprinkle vegetables with linguine shrimp, water for cooking pasta, lemon peel, and parsley.

Nutrition: 243 Calories 16g Fat 12g Protein

Brussels Sprout & Basil Bowties

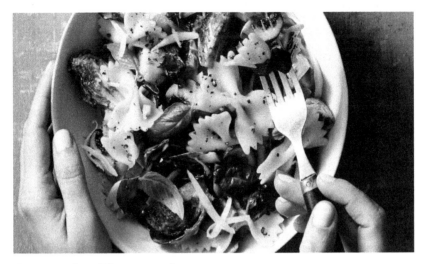

Preparation Time: 2 minutes

Cooking Time: 10 minutes

Servings: 4 - 6

Ingredients:

- 1/4 c. extra-virgin olive oil
- 3 cloves garlic, finely chopped
- 1/2 tsp. Kosher salt
- 1/2 lb. sliced onion
- 1/2 lb. sliced mushrooms
- 1/2 lb. chopped Brussels sprouts
- 1 tsp. finely chopped rosemary
- 1 lb. cooked bowtie pasta
- 1/2 c. reserved pasta cooking water
- 1/4 c. shredded Gruyere
- lemon juice

- Fresh basil
- Freshly ground black pepper

Directions:

1. Heat olive oil and garlic over medium for 3 minutes in a deep 12 "skillet, stirring.
2. Add salt, onion, mushrooms, and sprouts from Brussels.
3. Cook 5 minutes. Add rosemary. Cook for 3 minutes.
4. Cook pasta according to the instructions for the package and reserve 1/2 cup of the cooking water.
5. Toss pasta, cooking water and vegetables with Gruyere.
6. Garnish with black pepper, basil and lemon juice.

Nutrition: 276 Calories 16g Fat 9g Protein

Balsamic Mushroom Pasta

Preparation Time: 10 minutes

Cooking Time: 25 minutes

Servings: 2

Ingredients:

- 4 ounces fettuccine pasta
- 2 tablespoons butter, divided
- 1 tablespoon olive oil
- 1/4 cup shallot, finely diced
- 2 garlic cloves, minced
- 8 ounces baby portobello mushrooms, sliced
- 1/4 cup balsamic vinegar
- 1/4 cup heavy cream
- 1 tablespoon fresh parsley, chopped
- 1/4 cup grated parmesan cheese
- 1/2 teaspoon salt
- 1/4 teaspoon pepper

Directions:

1. Cook the fettuccine according to product directions.
2. Cook 1 tablespoon of butter over medium heat in a wide saucepan with 1 tablespoon of olive oil.
3. When cooled, add the shallots and garlic, and cook until softened for a few minutes or so. Add the sliced champignons and stir them to cover them with butter and olive oil.

---

4. If required, add an extra spoonful of olive oil if the mushrooms get too dry. Let them cook for about 8 minutes, and brown it.

5. Pour the balsamic vinegar into the pan and stir it together.

6. Add the other butter spoonful. Cook everything for a few minutes, then switch off the heat and push the pan off the burner.

7. Pour in the parmesan cheese and cream, and stir to combine. Add the cooked fettuccine to the sauce and combine to toss.

8. Stir in the new parsley, season with salt and pepper. Sprinkle parmesan cheese over the top.

Nutrition: 243 Calories 16g Fat 5g Protein

Spaghetti with No-Cook Heirloom Tomato Sauce

Preparation Time: 15 minutes

Cooking Time: 20 minutes

Servings: 4

Ingredients:

- 1 lb. heirloom plum tomatoes (about 5)
- 1/4 c. extra virgin olive oil
- Kosher salt and black pepper
- 12 oz. whole-wheat spaghetti
- 2 cloves garlic, crushed
- 3/4 tsp. crushed red pepper
- 1/4 c. roasted almonds, coarsely chopped
- 1/4 c. chopped fresh basil
- 2 tbsp. chopped fresh parsley
- 1 oz. ricotta Salata, shaved with a peeler (about 1/2 c.)

Directions:

1. Chop 4 tomatoes thinly; move to broad olive oil bowl and 1/4 teaspoon salt.
2. As the label tells, Cook spaghetti. Reserve 1/4 cup water to cook; drain pasta.
3. Chop remaining tomatoes, meanwhile. Place with garlic, red pepper, 3 tablespoons of almonds and 1/2 teaspoon of salt in the food processor; purée until smooth.

4. Remove the tomatoes into a bowl. Add cooked spaghetti, basil and parsley; toss, if necessary, add some reserved water for pasta.

5. Divide pasta between bowls to serve. Top with remaining almonds and cheese.

Nutrition: 266 Calories 13g Fat 16g Carbohydrates

MAIN RECIPES

Ramen Bowl

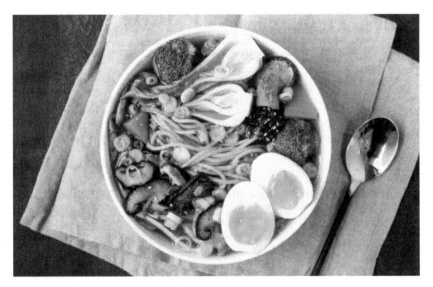

Preparation Time: 10 minutes

Cooking Time: 20 minutes

Servings: 4

Ingredients:

- 12 oz of pork belly, cut into ¼" chunks

- 1 tbsp of minced garlic

- 2 tsps. of grated ginger

- 4 cups of broth/water

- 3 tbsps. of coconut aminos

- 2 tsps. of chili flakes
- 2 tbsps. of sesame seeds
- 1 tbsp of soy sauce
- 1 tsp of paprika
- salt & pepper to taste
- 2 cups of mushrooms, thinly sliced
- 10 oz of zucchini noodles
- 3 soft boiled eggs, halved
- 6 scallops, chopped fine
- 4 sheets of seaweed

Directions:

1. Prepare the pork belly: place it in a large, deep-set pan over medium-high heat. Drizzle in a small amount of oil if necessary and cook the pork belly for 5 minutes on either side, until brown and crispy.

2. Remove the pork belly from the pan and set aside, leave the fat in the pan.

3. Reduce the heat to a medium-low and add the ginger and garlic into the pan. Stir the contents for about 1 minute until fragrant.

4. Pour the broth, coconut aminos, chili flakes, mushrooms, soy sauce, paprika, and a pinch of salt and pepper into the pan. Raise the temperature to a boil, then reduce the heat to a simmer. Allow the contents to simmer for about 10 minutes, stirring regularly.

5. Lastly, add the zucchini noodles into the pan and cook for another 5 minutes.

6. Spoon the ramen into bowls and add a few chunks of pork belly, an egg, and a seaweed sheet. Garnish with a few chopped scallops and sesame seeds.

Nutrition 595 Calories 30g Fat 60g Protein

Chipotle® Chicken

Preparation Time: 10 minutes

Cooking Time: 20 minutes

Servings: 8

Ingredients:

- 2 1/2 pound organic boneless and skinless chicken breasts or thighs
- Olive oil or cooking spray

Marinade

- 7 oz. chipotle peppers in adobo sauce
- 2 tablespoons olive oil
- 6 garlic cloves, peeled
- 1 teaspoon black pepper
- 2 teaspoons salt
- 1/2 teaspoon cumin
- 1/2 teaspoon dry oregano

Directions:

1. Pour all the marinade ingredients in a food processor or blender and blend until you get a smooth paste.
2. Pound the chicken until it has a thickness between 1/2 to ¾ inch. Place chicken into an airtight container or re-sealable plastic bag such as a Ziploc. Pour the marinade over the chicken and stir until well coated. Place the chicken in the refrigerator and let marinate overnight or up to 24 hours.

3. Pour the blended mixture into the container and marinate the chicken for at least 8 hours.

4. Cook the chicken over medium to high heat on an oiled and preheated grill for 3 to 5 minutes per side. The internal temperature of the chicken should be 165 Fahrenheit before you remove it from the heat. You can also cook it in a heavy-bottomed skillet over medium heat with a little olive oil.

5. Let rest before serving. If desired, cut into cubes to add to salads, tacos, or quesadillas or serve as is.

Nutrition: Calories 293, Fat 18.7 g, Carbs 5.8 g, Protein 24.9 g,

Longhorns® Parmesan Crusted Chicken

Preparation Time: 10 minutes

Cooking Time: 30 minutes

Servings: 4

Ingredients:

- 4 chicken breasts, skinless
- 2 teaspoons salt
- 2 teaspoons ground black pepper
- 2 tablespoons avocado oil

For the Marinade:

- 1 tablespoon minced garlic
- 1/2 teaspoon ground black pepper
- 1 teaspoon juice
- 3 tablespoon Worcester sauce
- 1 teaspoon white vinegar
- 1/2 cup avocado oil
- 1/2 cup ranch dressing

For the Parmesan Crust:

- 1 cup panko breadcrumbs 6 ounces parmesan cheese, chopped
- 5 tablespoons melted butter, unsalted
- 6 ounces provolone cheese, chopped
- 2 teaspoons garlic powder
- 6 tablespoons ranch dressing, low-carb

Directions:

1. Prepare the marinade and for this, take a little bowl, place all of its ingredients in it then whisk until well combined. Pound each chicken until ¾-inch thick, then season with salt and black pepper and transfer chicken pieces to an outsized bag.

2. Pour within the prepared marinade, seal the bag, turn it upside to coat chicken with it and let it rest for a minimum of half-hour within the refrigerator.

3. Then take an outsized skillet pan, place it over medium-high heat, add oil and when hot, place marinated pigeon breast in it then cook for five minutes per side until chicken is not any longer pink and nicely seared on all sides.

4. Transfer chicken to a plate and repeat it with the remaining chicken pieces. Meanwhile, turn on the oven, set it to 450 degrees F, and let it preheat.

5. When the chicken has cooked, prepare the parmesan crust and for this, take a little heatproof bowl, place both cheeses in it, pour in ranch dressing and milk, stir until mixed, then microwave for 30 seconds. Then stir the cheese mixture again until smooth and continue microwaving for an additional 15 seconds.

6. Stir the cheese mixture again, spread evenly on top of every pigeon breast, arrange them during a baking sheet then bake for five minutes until cheese has melted.

7. Meanwhile, take a little bowl, place breadcrumbs in it, stir in garlic powder and butter in it. After 5 minutes of baking, spread the breadcrumbs mixture on top of the chicken then continue baking for two minutes until the panko mixture turns brown. Serve chicken immediately with cauliflower mashed potatoes.

Nutrition: Calories 557; Fats 42g; Protein 31g; Carb 10g

Carrabba® Pollo Rosa Maria

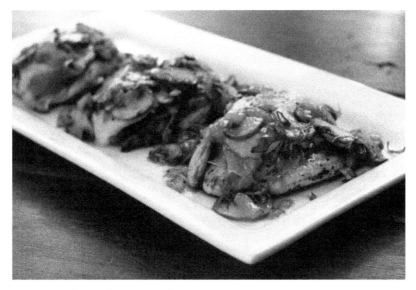

Preparation Time: 5 minutes

Cooking Time: 50 minutes

Servings: 4

Ingredients:

- 4 butterflied chicken breasts
- 4 slices prosciutto
- 4 slices Fontina cheese
- 1/2 cup clarified butter
- 3 garlic cloves
- 1/2 sweet onion, diced
- 1/4 cup dry white wine
- 4 tablespoons unsalted butter
- 1/2 white pepper
- 1 dash salt

- 8 ounces cremini mushrooms, sliced
- 1/2 cup fresh basil, chopped
- 1 lemon, juiced
- Shredded Parmesan for garnish

Directions:

1. Grill the chicken breasts on each side for 3 to 5 minutes.
2. Remove the chicken from heat and then stuff with the prosciutto and cheese. Place the ham and cheese on one side of the chicken and fold it over. Secure the filling with a toothpick.
3. Wrap the chicken in foil to keep it warm.
4. Sauté the onions and garlic in butter until they become tender. Add the white wine to deglaze the pan.
5. In the same pan, sauté the mushrooms in the salt, pepper, and butter until tender, then add the remaining ingredients and cook until completely blended.
6. Transfer the chicken to a plate and pour the mushroom sauce over it. Remove the toothpick and serve. Garnish with Parmesan cheese, if desired

Nutrition: Calories 644.4, Fat 52.3 g, Carbs 6 g, Protein 36 g

Panda Express® Kung Pao Chicken

Preparation Time: 10 minutes

Cooking Time: 30 minutes

Servings: 10

Ingredients:

- 35 ounces chicken thighs, skinless
- 1/2-inch cubed 14 ounces zucchini, destemmed
- 1/2-inch diced 14 ounces red bell pepper, cored
- 1-inch cubed 1 scallion, sliced
- 15 pieces of dried Chinese red peppers
- 1 1/2 teaspoons minced garlic
- 1 teaspoon minced ginger
- 3 ounces roasted peanuts
- 1/4 teaspoon ground black pepper
- 1/4 teaspoon xanthan gum
- 3 tablespoons copra oil
- 1 tablespoon balsamic vinegar
- 1 tablespoon chili aioli
- ¾ tablespoon vegetable oil

For the Marinade:

- 3 tablespoons coconut aminos
- 1 tablespoon copra oil
- For the Sauce:
- 3 tablespoons monk fruit sweetener

- 3 tablespoons coconut aminos

Directions:

1. Marinade the chicken and for this, take an outsized bowl, place the chicken pieces in it, then add all the ingredients for the marinade in it. Stir until chicken is well coated then marinate for a minimum of half-hour within the refrigerator.

2. Then take an outsized skillet pan, add 1 tablespoon of copra oil in it and when it melted, add marinated chicken and cook for 10 minutes or more until it starts to release its water.

3. After 10 minutes, push the chicken to the edges of the pan to make a well in its middle, slowly stir in xanthan gum into the water released by chicken and cook for two to 4 minutes until it starts to thicken.

4. Then stir chicken into the thicken liquid and continue cooking for 10 minutes or more until chicken has thoroughly cooked, put aside until required. Return pan over medium-high heat, add 1 tablespoon oil, and when it melts, add bell pepper and zucchini cubes then cook for five to eight minutes until lightly browned.

5. Transfer vegetables to a separate plate, then add remaining copra oil into the pan, add Chinese red peppers, ginger, garlic, vinegar, and chili aioli. Stir until mixed, cook for 3 minutes, add ingredients for the sauce alongside peanuts, scallion, black pepper, and

vegetable oil and continue cooking for 3 minutes, stirring frequently. Return chicken and vegetables into the pan, toss until well mixed then continue cooking for 3 to five minutes until hot. Serve immediately.

Nutrition: Calories 295; Fats 16.4g; Protein 31.7g; Carb 3.2g

Olive Garden® Parmesan Crusted Chicken

Preparation Time: 15 minutes

Cooking Time: 40 minutes

Servings: **4**

Ingredients:

Breading

- 1 cup plain breadcrumbs
- 2 tablespoons flour
- 1/4 cup grated parmesan cheese

For dipping

- 1 cup milk
- Chicken
- 2 chicken breasts
- Vegetable oil for frying
- 2 cups cooked linguini pasta
- 2 tablespoons butter
- 3 tablespoons olive oil
- 2 teaspoons crushed garlic
- 1/2 cup white wine
- 1/4 cup water
- 2 tablespoons flour
- ¾ cup half-and-half
- 1/4 cup sour cream

- 1/2 teaspoon salt
- 1 teaspoon fresh flat leave parsley, finely diced¾ cup mild Asiago cheese, finely grated
- Garnish
- 1 Roma tomato, diced
- Grated parmesan cheese
- Fresh flat-leaf parsley, finely chopped

Directions:

1. Pound the chicken until it flattens to 1/2 inch thick.
2. Mix the breading ingredients in one shallow bowl and place the milk in another.
3. Heat some oil over medium to medium-to-low heat.
4. Dip the chicken in the breading, then the milk, then the breading again. Immediately place into the heated oil.
5. Cook the chicken in the oil until golden brown, about 3-4 minutes per side. Remove the chicken and set aside on a plate lined with paper towels.
6. Create a roux by adding flour to heated olive oil and butter over medium heat.
7. When the roux is done, add the garlic, water, and salt to the pan and stir.
8. Add the wine and continue stirring and cooking.
9. Add the half-and-half and sour cream and stir some more.
10. Add the cheese and let it melt.

11. Finally, add in the parsley and remove from heat. Add pasta and stir to coat.

12. Divide the hot pasta between serving plates.

13. Top each dish with the chicken, diced tomatoes, and parmesan cheese before serving.

Nutrition: Calories 595, Fat 41g, Carbs 35g, Protein 12g

Olive Garden® Chicken Marsala

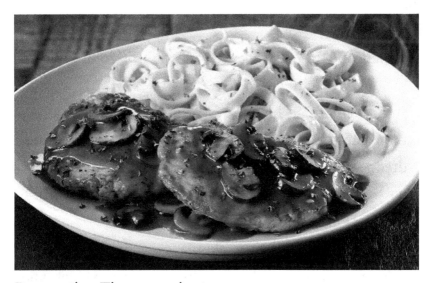

Preparation Time: 10 minutes

Cooking Time: 40 minutes

Servings: 4-6

Ingredients:

- 2 tablespoons olive oil
- 2 tablespoons butter
- 4 boneless skinless chicken breasts
- 1 1/2 cups sliced mushrooms
- 1 small clove garlic, thinly sliced

Flour for dredging

- Sea salt and freshly ground black pepper
- 1 1/2 cups chicken stock
- 1 1/2 cups Marsala wine
- 1 tablespoon lemon juice

- 1 teaspoon Dijon mustard

Directions:

Chicken scaloppini:

1. Pound out the chicken with a mallet or rolling pin to about 1/2 inch thick

2. In a large skillet, heat the olive oil and 1 tablespoon of the butter over medium-high heat. When the oil is hot, dredge the chicken in flour. Season with salt and pepper on both sides. Dredge only as many as will fit in the skillet. Don't overcrowd the pan.

3. Cook chicken in batches, about 1 to 2 minutes on each side or until cooked through. Remove from skillet, and place on an oven-proof platter. Keep warm, in the oven, while the rest of the chicken is cooking.

Marsala sauce:

4. In the same skillet, add 1 tablespoon of olive oil. On medium-high heat, sauté mushrooms and garlic until softened. Remove the mushrooms from the pan and set aside.

5. Add the chicken stock and loosen any remaining bits in the pan. On high heat, let reduce by half, about 6-8 minutes. Add Marsala wine and lemon juice and in the same manner reduce by half, about 6-8 minutes. Add the mushroom back in the saucepan, and stir in the Dijon mustard. Warm for 1 minute on medium-low heat. Remove from heat, stir in the remaining butter to

make the sauce silkier. To serve, pour the sauce over chicken, and serve immediately.

Nutrition: Calories 970, Fat 43g, Carbs 71g, Protein 66g

KFC® Fried Chicken

Preparation Time: 15 minutes

Cooking Time: 18 minutes

Servings: 6

Ingredients:

For the Seasoning:

- 1 teaspoon flavored
- 1 teaspoon of sea salt
- 1 teaspoon ginger powder
- 1 tablespoon ground white pepper
- 2 teaspoons flavored
- 1 teaspoon ground black pepper
- 4 teaspoons paprika
- 1/4 teaspoon dried oregano
- 1/2 teaspoon dried thyme
- 1 teaspoon mustard powder

For the Marinade:

- 1/2 of the seasoning
- 4 tablespoons white vinegar
- 3 tablespoons cream 2 cups almond milk, unsweetened
- 2 eggs

For the Chicken:

- 8 1/2 cups avocado oil
- 2 pounds of chicken drumsticks
- 2 1/2 cups whey protein powder

Directions:

1. Prepare the seasoning and for this, take a little bowl, place all of its ingredients in it then stir until mixed, put aside until required. Prepare the marinade and for this, take an outsized bowl, pour in milk, add vinegar and cream, whisk until blended then let it sit for 10 minutes.

2. Then whisk in eggs until combined, and whisk in 1/2 of seasoning until smooth. Place chicken pieces into an outsized bag, pour within the marinade, seal the bag, turn it the wrong way up to coat chicken then let it marinate within the refrigerator for a minimum of 4 hours.

3. Cook the chicken, and for this, take an outsized pan, place it over medium heat, pour within the oil, and warmth it for 12 minutes or more until the temperature reaches 325 degrees F. Spread remaining seasoning mixture on a plate, take a chicken piece, coat it with the seasoning mix then add into the pan.

4. Add more seasoned chicken pieces into the pan until filled and cook for 16 to 18 minutes until the interior temperature of chicken reaches 165 degrees F and turns nicely browned, turning chicken frequently. When done, transfer fried chicken to a plate lined with paper towels, then repeat with the remaining chicken pieces. Serve immediately.

Nutrition: Calories 590.2; Fats 39.6g; Protein 57.6 g; Carb 1.1g

Addy's Bar and Grill® Buffalo wings

Cooking Time: 45 minutes

Preparation Time: 10 minutes

Servings: 3

Ingredients:

- 12 chicken wings, frozen
- 1/2 teaspoon salt
- 1/4 teaspoon ground black pepper
- 1/2 cup avocado oil

For the Sauce:

- 1/2 tablespoon minced garlic
- 1/4 teaspoon paprika
- 1/4 teaspoon cayenne pepper
- 4 tablespoons butter, salted
- 1/4 cup sauce, low-carb

Directions:

1. Switch on the oven, then set it to 400 degrees F and let it preheat. Meanwhile, take an outsized baking dish, spread chicken wings thereon, rub them with oil, and then sprinkle with salt and black pepper.

2. Bake the chicken wings for 45 minutes until crisp, turning halfway through. Meanwhile, prepare the sauce and for this, take a little saucepan, place it over medium-low heat, add butter and garlic and cook for 3 to five minutes until butter melts.

3. Add remaining ingredients for the sauce, whisk until combined, cook for two minutes until hot, and then remove pan from heat. Add baked chicken wings into the sauce then toss until well coated. Serve immediately.

Nutrition: Calories 391; Fats 32g; Protein 31g; Carb 1g

Tso® Chicken

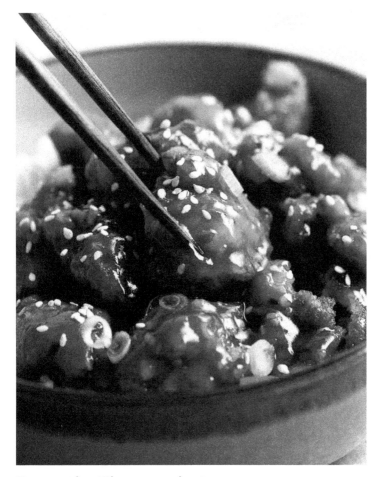

Preparation Time: 10 minutes

Cooking Time: 20 minutes

Servings: 4

Ingredients:

For the Chicken:

- 1 1/2 pounds chicken thighs, boneless

- 1 scallion, chopped
- 1/2 cup almond flour
- 1/4 teaspoon salt
- 1/4 teaspoon ground black pepper
- 1/2 teaspoon xanthan gum
- 2 egg whites
- 2 tablespoons copra oil
- 1/2 cup chicken stock
- 1 teaspoon sesame seeds For the Sauce:
- 1 1/2 tablespoon minced garlic
- 1/2 teaspoon grated ginger
- 1 teaspoon Swerve sweetener
- 1 teaspoon red chili paste
- 5 tablespoons soy
- 2 tablespoons ketchup, sugar-free
- 1 teaspoon vegetable oil

Directions:

1. Prepare the sauce and for this, take a medium bowl, place all of its ingredients in it then whisk until combined, put aside until required. Prepare the chicken and for this, cut it into bite-size pieces then season it with salt and black pepper.

2. Take a shallow dish, crack the egg in it and whisk until frothy. Take a separate shallow dish then spread flour in it. Working on one chicken piece at a time, first dip it

into the egg, dredge it into the flour until coated, and repeat with the remaining pieces.

3. Plug-in the moment pot, press the 'sauté' button, add oil and when hot, add chicken pieces during a single layer then cook them for 3 to 4 minutes per side until golden brown.

4. Transfer the chicken pieces to a plate and repeat with the remaining chicken pieces. When done, stir broth into the inner pot to get rid of browned bits from rock bottom of the pot, return chicken pieces into the pot and pour the prepared sauce over them.

5. Shut the moment pot with its lid within the sealed position, press the manual button, and let the chicken cook for 4 minutes. When the moment pot, do a fast pressure release, then open the moment pot and stir xanthan gum into the chicken until sauce thickens. Top chicken with sesame seeds and green onions and serve with cauliflower rice.

Nutrition: Calories 427; Fats 30g; Protein 35g; Carb 1g

Applebee® Fiesta Lime Chicken

Preparation Time: 10 minutes

Cooking Time: 13 minutes

Servings: 4

Ingredients:

- 1 pound pigeon breast
- 1 cup shredded Colby-Monterey jack cheese For the Marinade:
- 1 1/2 teaspoon minced garlic
- 1/4 teaspoon ginger powder
- 1/2 teaspoon salt
- 1 teaspoon liquid smoke
- 1/2 of lime, juiced
- 1/3 cup teriyaki sauce
- 1 teaspoon tequila
- 1 cup of water

For the Dressing:

- 1 teaspoon Cajun spice mix
- 1/4 teaspoon dried parsley
- 1/8 teaspoon cumin
- 1/8 teaspoon dried dill
- 1/4 teaspoon sauce
- 2 tablespoons spicy salsa, low-carb
- 1 tablespoon coconut milk, unsweetened

- 1/4 cup soured cream
- 1/4 cup mayonnaise

Directions:

1. Prepare the marinade and for this, take an outsized bowl, place all of its ingredients in it then whisk until combined. Add chicken, toss until well coated then let the chicken marinate within the refrigerator for a minimum of two hours.

2. Meanwhile, prepare the dressing and for this, take an outsized bowl, place all of its ingredients in it, whisk until combined, and let it rest within the refrigerator until chilled.

3. When the chicken has marinated, found out the grill and let it preheat at a high heat setting for five minutes.

4. Place chicken on the cooking grate then cook it for five minutes per side until thoroughly cooked.

5. When done, brush the chicken generously with prepared dressing, arrange chicken during a baking sheet, and sprinkle cheese on top, then broil for 3 minutes until cheese has melted.

6. Serve chicken immediately.

Nutrition: Calories 294; Fat 14.5g; Protein 33.2g; Carb 6.1g

Garcia® Pollo Fundido

Preparation Time: 10 minutes

Cooking Time: 45 minutes

Servings: 4

Ingredients:

- 2 pounds of chicken breasts
- 4 ounces diced green chilies
- 1/2 teaspoon garlic powder
- 1/4 teaspoon of sea salt
- 1/4 teaspoon ground black pepper
- 1/4 teaspoon cumin
- 8 ounces cheese, softened
- 1 cup Monterrey jack cheese

Directions:

1. Switch on the oven, then set it to 375 degrees F and let it preheat. Meanwhile, take an outsized bowl, place cheese in it, add all the seasoning and spices, stir well until well combined, and then fold within the green chilies until incorporated.

2. Take an outsized baking dish, place chicken breasts in it with some space between them, and spread cheese mixture on the highest evenly. Sprinkle cheese on the highest then bake for 45 minutes until the chicken has thoroughly cooked. When done, let the chicken cool for five minutes then serve.

Nutrition: Calories 520; Fats 25g; Protein 62g; Carb 5g

Popeye® Chicken Strips

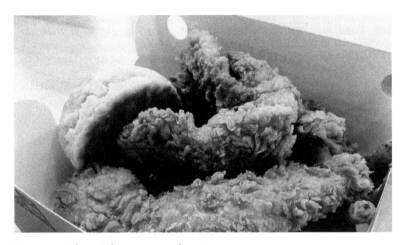

Preparation Time: 10 minutes

Cooking Time: 20 minutes

Servings: 6

Ingredients:

- 2 pounds of chicken breasts
- 2/3 cup almond flour
- 2 teaspoons salt
- 1 teaspoon chipotle flavored
- 2 teaspoons smoked paprika
- 1/3 cup Louisiana style sauce, low-carb 3 eggs
- 1/2 cup almond milk, unsweetened
- Avocado oil as required for frying

Directions:

1. Take a little bowl, pour within the milk, and then whisk in sauce. Cut each pigeon breast into four strips, place

them into an outsized bowl, pour in half the milk mixture, and then marinate for a minimum of 1 hour.

2. Then take a shallow dish, place flour in it, and stir in salt, paprika, and chipotle until mixed. Crack the eggs into the remaining milk mixture then whisk until frothy.

3. When the chicken has marinated, drain it well, dredge each chicken strip into the flour mixture, read the egg mixture and dredge again in flour mixture. When able to cook, take an outsized skillet pan, fill it 2 1/2-inches of oil, place the pan over medium-high heat and convey the oil to 360 degrees F.

4. Then lower the chicken pieces into the oil, don't overcrowd it, and then cook for five to 7 minutes per side until cooked and golden brown. Transfer chicken pieces to a plate lined with paper towels then repeat with the remaining chicken pieces. Serve immediately.

Nutrition: Calories 385; Fats 25g; Protein 35g; Carb 4g

Olive Garden® Chicken Piccata

Preparation Time: 10 minutes

Cooking Time: 15 minutes

Servings: 5

Ingredients:

- 2 pounds chicken breasts, thinly sliced
- 2 tablespoons chopped parsley
- 1/4 cup drained capers, rinsed
- 1/2 teaspoon salt
- 1/2 teaspoon ground black pepper
- 1/3 cup juice
- 2 tablespoons avocado oil
- 4 tablespoons butter, unsalted, divided
- 1/2 cup chicken stock

Directions:

1. Prepare the chicken and for this, pound the chicken with a meat mallet then season with salt and black pepper.

2. Take an outsized skillet pan, place it over medium-high heat, add oil and a couple of tablespoons of butter and when hot, add chicken until the pan is filled then cook for two minutes per side until nicely golden brown.

3. When done, transfer chicken to a plate then repeats with the remaining chicken.

4. When done, stir juice and broth into the pan to get rid of browned bits from the pan, add capers then bring the mixture to a boil.

5. Return chicken into the pan, simmer for two minutes, and then transfer chicken pieces to a plate.

6. Add remaining butter into the pan, whisk it until combined, then drizzle the sauce over chicken. Garnish the chicken with parsley then serve.

Nutrition: Calories 309; Fat15g; Protein 43g; Carb 0.3g

Cheesecake Factory® Tuna Tataki Salad

Preparation Time: 10 minutes

Cooking Time: 5 minutes

Servings: 4

Ingredients:

For the Tuna:

- 1 pound tuna, sashimi grade
- 4 tablespoons avocado oil

For the Salad:

- 4 radishes, peeled, sliced thinly
- 8 cups salad greens
- 4 green onion, sliced
- 4 avocados, peeled, pitted, sliced
- 2 teaspoons black sesame seeds

For the Salad Dressing:

- 2 1-inch pieces of ginger, grated
- 2 tablespoons liquid stevia
- 4 tablespoons ponzu sauce, low-carb
- 2 tablespoons sake
- 2 tablespoons soy sauce
- 2 tablespoons toasted sesame oil

Directions:

1. Prepare the salad dressing and for this, take a mason jar, place all of its ingredients in it, shut with the lid,

and then shake well until well blended, set aside until required.

2. Take a large salad bowl, place avocado slices, radish, and salad greens in it, and then toss until mixed. Prepare the tuna and for this, take a large skillet pan, place it over medium heat, add oil and when hot, add tuna and then cook for 1 minute per side until seared.

3. Transfer tuna to a plate, repeat with the remaining tuna, let cool for 15 minutes and then cut tuna into thin slices. Distribute salad evenly among four plates, add seared tuna to the side and then drizzle with prepared salad dressing. Sprinkle sesame seeds and green onion over tuna and then serve.

Nutrition: Calories 594; Fat 42.2g; Protein 37.1g; Carb 4.4g

Outback Steakhouse® Coconut Shrimp

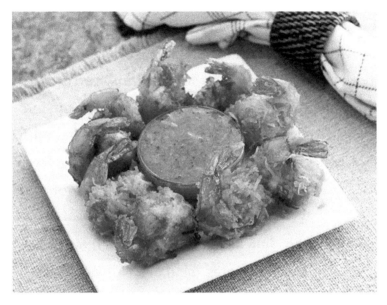

Cooking Time: 14 minutes

Preparation Time: 10 minutes

Servings: 4

Ingredients:

- 1-pound medium shrimp, tail removed, peeled, deveined, cooked
- 1/2 cup pork rind
- 1 teaspoon salt
- 1/2 cup shredded coconut, unsweetened
- 1/2 teaspoon ground black pepper
- 1/4 cup coconut milk, unsweetened

Directions:

1. Take a shallow pan, place it over low heat and when hot, add coconut and cook for 3 to 4 minutes until golden brown. Take a shallow dish, and then pour in the milk. Take a separate shallow dish, place coconut and pork rind in it, and then stir until mixed. Pat dries the shrimp with paper towels then dip each shrimp into milk and dredge in the pork-coconut mixture until evenly coated. Plugin the air fryer, insert a greased fryer basket, set it 400 degrees F, and let it preheat for 400 degrees F.

2. Then add shrimps in a single layer into the fryer basket and then fry for 7 minutes, shaking halfway. When done, transfer fried shrimps to a plate and repeat with the remaining shrimps. Season the shrimps with salt and black pepper and then serve.

Nutrition: Calories 335; Fat15.6g; Protein 46.1g; Carb 0.9g

Cheesecake Factory® Bang Bang Shrimp

Preparation Time: 10 minutes

Cooking Time: 12 minutes

Servings: 4

Ingredients:

For the Shrimp:

- 1 pound shrimp, tail removed, peeled, deveined
- 1/2 cup coconut flour
- Avocado oil as needed for frying
- 1 scallion, sliced

For the Sauce:

- 1/3 cup mayonnaise
- 1 ¾ tablespoon garlic chili sauce
- 1 1/2 tablespoon rice vinegar
- 2 1/2 tablespoons monk fruit Sweetener
- 1/8 teaspoon salt

Directions:

1. Prepare the shrimps and for this, dredge each shrimp in coconut flour and then arrange on a baking sheet. Then take a large skillet pan, place it over medium-high heat, fill it 2-inch with oil and when hot, add shrimps in it and then cook for 4 minutes or more until pink.

2. When done, transfer shrimps to a plate lined with paper towels and repeat with the remaining shrimps. Prepare

the sauce and for this, plug in a food processor, add all the ingredients in it, cover with the lid and then pulse for 30 seconds until smooth.

3. Tip the sauce into a large bowl, add shrimps and then toss until coated. Garnish shrimps with scallion and then serve.

Nutrition: Calories 204; Fat16g; Protein 20g; Carb 3g

Dockside Grill Restaurant® Fish Cakes

Cooking Time: 16 minutes

Preparation Time: 5 minutes

Servings: 2

Ingredients:

For the Fish Cake:

- 1-pound white fish, boneless
- 1/4 cup cilantro leaves
- 1/4 teaspoon salt
- 1/4 teaspoon red chili flakes
- 1 tablespoon minced garlic
- 2 tablespoons avocado oil

For the Dip:

- 1 lemon, juiced
- 2 avocados, peeled, pitted
- 1/4 teaspoon salt
- 2 tablespoons water

Directions:

1. Prepare the fish cakes and for this, place all of its ingredients in a food processor except for oil and then pulse for 3 minutes until well combined.

2. Tip the mixture in a large bowl and then shape it into six patties.

3. Take a frying pan, place it over medium-high heat, add oil and when hot, add fish patties in it and then cook for 3 to 4 minutes per side until cooked and golden brown.

4. Meanwhile, prepare the dip and for this, place all of its ingredients in a food processor and then pulse for 2 minutes until smooth.

5. Serve fish cakes with prepared dip.

Nutrition: Calories 175; Fats 9.7g; Protein 9.1g; Carb 13g

APPETIZER RECIPES

Pei Wei® Thai Chicken Satay

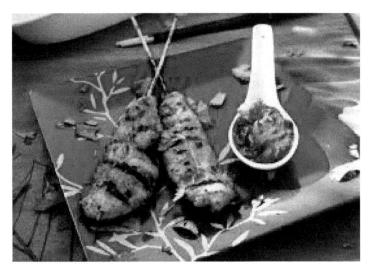

Preparation Time: 20 minutes

Cooking Time: 10-20 minutes

Servings: 2-4

Ingredients:

- 1-pound boneless, skinless chicken thighs
- 6-inch bamboo skewers, soaked in water
- Thai satay marinade
- 1 tablespoon coriander seeds
- 1 teaspoon cumin seeds

- 2 teaspoons chopped lemongrass
- 1 teaspoon salt
- 1 teaspoon turmeric powder
- 1/4 teaspoon roasted chili
- 1/2 cup coconut milk
- 1 1/2 tablespoons light brown sugar
- 1 teaspoon lime juice
- 2 teaspoons fish sauce
- Peanut sauce
- 2 tablespoons soy sauce
- 1 tablespoon rice wine vinegar
- 2 tablespoons brown sugar
- 1/4 cup peanut butter
- 1 teaspoon chipotle Tabasco

*Whisk all ingredients until well incorporated. Store in airtight container in the refrigerator and last for 3 days

- Thai sweet cucumber relish
- 1/4 cup white vinegar
- ¾ cup sugar
- ¾ cup water
- 1 tablespoon ginger, minced
- 1 Thai red chili, minced
- 1 medium cucumber
- 1 tablespoon toasted peanuts, chopped

Directions:

1. Cut any excess fat from the chicken, and then cut into strips about 3 inches long and 1 inch wide. Thread the strips onto the skewers.

2. Prepare the Thai Satay Marinade and the Peanut Sauce in separate bowls by simply whisking together all of the ingredients for each.

3. Dip the chicken skewers in the Thai Satay Marinade and allow to marinate for at least 4 hours. Reserve the marinade when you remove the chicken skewers.

4. You can either cook the skewers on the grill, basting with the marinade halfway through, or you can do the same in a 350-degree F oven. They taste better on the grill.

5. To prepare the Cucumber Relish, simply add all of the ingredients together and stir to make sure the cucumber is coated.

6. When the chicken skewers are done cooking, serve it with peanut sauce and the cucumber relish.

Nutrition: Calories 298; Fat 5.4g; Carbs 7.5g; Protein 61g

Pei Wei® Vietnamese Chicken Salad Spring Roll

Preparation Time: 10 minutes

Cooking Time: 1 minutes

Servings: 4-6

Ingredients:

Salad

- Rice Wrappers
- Green leaf lettuce like Boston Bibb lettuce
- Napa cabbage, shredded
- Green onions, chopped
- Mint, chopped
- Carrots cut into 1-inch matchsticks
- Peanuts
- Chicken, diced and cooked, about 6 chicken tenders drizzled with soy sauce, honey, garlic powder, and red pepper flakes

Lime dressing

- 2 tablespoons lime juice, about 1 lime
- 1 1/2 teaspoons water
- 1 tablespoon sugar
- 1 teaspoon salt
- Dash of pepper
- 3 tablespoons oil

Add everything but the oil to a small container or bowl and shake or stir until the sugar and salt are dissolved. Next, add the oil and shake well.

Peanut dipping sauce

- 2 tablespoons soy sauce
- 1 tablespoon rice wine vinegar
- 2 tablespoons brown sugar
- 1/4 cup peanut butter
- 1 teaspoon chipotle Tabasco
- 1 teaspoon honey
- 1 teaspoon sweet chili sauce
- 1 teaspoon lime vinaigrette

Mix all the ingredients to combine thoroughly in a small bowl

Directions:

1. In a large bowl, mix together all of the salad ingredients except for the rice wrappers and lettuce. Place the rice wrappers in warm water for about 1 minute to soften. Transfer the wrappers to a plate and top each with 2 pieces of lettuce.
2. Top the lettuce with the salad mixture and drizzle with the lime dressing. Fold the wrapper by tucking in the ends and then rolling. Serve with lime dressing and peanut dipping sauce.

Nutrition: Calories410; Fat 26g; Carbs 57g; Protein 39g

Chinese Restaurant® Dry Garlic Ribs

Preparation Time: 15 minutes

Cooking Time: 2 hours and 15 minutes

Servings: 4-6

Ingredients:

- 6 pounds pork ribs, silver skin removed and cut into individual ribs
- 1 1/2 cups broth
- 1 1/2 cups brown sugar
- 1/4 cup soy sauce
- 12 cloves garlic, minced
- 1/4 cup yellow mustard
- 1 large onion, finely chopped
- 1/4 teaspoon salt
- 1/2 teaspoon black pepper

Directions:

1. Preheat oven to 200°F. Season ribs with salt and pepper. Place it on a baking tray and then cover with aluminum foil.

2. Bake for 1 hour. In a mixing bowl, stir together the broth, brown sugar, soy sauce, garlic, mustard and onion. Continue stirring until the sugar is completely dissolved.

3. After an hour, remove the foil from the ribs and turn the heat up to 350°F.Carefully pour the sauce over the ribs. Cover with foil again and then return to the oven for 1 hour. Remove the foil and bake for 15 more minutes on each side.

Nutrition: Calories 233; Fat 3.6g; Carbs 6.4g; Protein 65g

Abuelo's Restaurant® Jalapeno Poppers

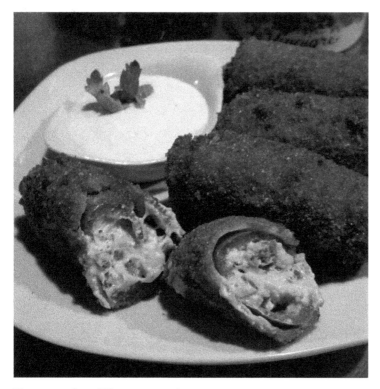

Preparation Time: 10 minutes

Cooking Time: 1 hour and 10 minutes

Servings: 8

Ingredients:

- 30 jalapeno peppers; sliced into half lengthwise
- 1 cup milk
- 2 packages soften cream cheese, at room temperature (8-ounces each)
- 1/8 teaspoon paprika

- 12 ounces Cheddar cheese, shredded
- 1/8 teaspoon chili powder
- 1 cup flour
- 1/8 teaspoon garlic powder
- 1 cup seasoned breadcrumbs
- 1/4 teaspoon ground black pepper
- 1 quart of oil for frying
- 1/4 teaspoon salt

Directions:

1. Scrape out seeds and the pith inside of the jalapeno peppers using a spoon. Combine cheddar cheese together with cream cheese in a medium-sized bowl; give them a good stir until blended well. Fill each pepper half with the prepared cream cheese blend using a spoon.

2. Add flour into a small-sized shallow bowl. Add paprika, pepper, garlic powder, chili powder and salt. Blend into the flour until it is mixed. Pour milk into a separate medium-sized shallow bowl. Dip stuffed jalapeno into flour. Place the floured pepper on a large-sized baking sheet with a rack. Let dry for 10 minutes.

3. Pour the dried breadcrumbs into a separate bowl. Dip the floured jalapeno pepper into the milk & then into the bowl with the breadcrumbs. Place the pepper on the rack again. Preheat the oil to 350 F in advance. Dip the pepper into the milk & then into the breadcrumbs.

4. Repeat these steps until you have utilized the entire dipping peppers. Work in batches and fry peppers for a minute or two, until turn golden brown. Remove from oil & place them on a baking rack to drain.

Nutrition: Calories 257; Fat 14.3g; Carbs 18.9g; Protein 21.5g

Applebee® Baja Potato Boats

Preparation Time: 10 minutes

Cooking Time: 30 minutes

Servings: 4

Ingredients:

For Pico de Gallo:

- 1 1/2 teaspoon fresh cilantro, minced
- 1 tablespoon canned jalapeño slices (nacho slices), diced
- 3 tablespoons Spanish onion, chopped
- 1 chopped tomato (approximately 1/2 cup)
- A dash each of freshly-ground black pepper & salt

For the Potato Boats:

- 2 slices Canadian bacon diced (roughly 2 tablespoons)
- Canola oil non-stick cooking spray, as required
- 1/3Cup Cheddar cheese, shredded
- 3 russet potatoes, medium
- 1/3Cup Mozzarella cheese
- Salt as needed

On the Side:

- Salsa & sour cream

Directions:

1. Combine the entire Pico De Gallo ingredients together in a large bowl; mix well. When done, place in a refrigerator until ready to use.

2. Preheat your oven to 400 F in advance. Place potatoes in oven & bake until tender, for an hour. Set aside at room temperature until easy to handle.

3. When done, cut them lengthwise 2 times. This should make 3 1/2 to ¾" slices, throwing the middle slices away.

4. Increase your oven's temperature to 450 F. Take a spoon & scoop out the inside of the potato skins. Ensure that you must leave at least 1/4 of an inch of the potato inside each skin.

5. Spray the potato skin completely on all sides with the spray of nonstick canola oil. Put the skins, cut-side facing up on a large-sized cookie sheet. Sprinkle them with salt & bake in the preheated oven until the edges start to turn brown, for 12 to 15 minutes.

6. Combine both the cheeses together in a large bowl. Sprinkle approximately 1 1/2 tablespoons of the mixture on each potato skin. Then sprinkle a teaspoon of the Canadian bacon over the cheese. Top this with a large tablespoon of the Pico de Gallo and then sprinkle each skin with some more of cheese.

7. Place the skins into the oven again & bake until the cheese melts, for 2 to 4 more minutes. Remove & let them sit for a minute. Slice each one lengthwise using a sharp knife.

8. Serve hot with some salsa and sour cream on the side.

Nutrition: Calories 254; Fat 24g; Carbs 43g; Protein 55g

Applebee® Chicken Wings

Preparation Time: 15 minutes

Cooking Time: 35 minutes

Servings: 6

Ingredients:

- 35 chicken wings
- 1 1/2 tablespoon flour
- 3 tablespoons vinegar
- 1 1/4 teaspoon cayenne pepper
- 1 tablespoon Worcestershire sauce
- 12 ounces Louisiana hot sauce
- 1/4 teaspoon garlic powder

Directions:

1. Cook the chicken wings either by deep-frying or baking. Mix the entire sauce ingredients (except the flour) together over low-medium heat in a large saucepan. Cook until warm and then add in the flour; stir well until you get your desired level of thickness.

2. When thick; cover the bottom of 9x13" baking dish with the sauce. Combine the leftover sauce with the cooked wings & place them in the baking dish. Bake until warm, for 15 to 20 minutes, at 300 F. Serve with blue-cheese dressing and celery sticks. Enjoy.

Nutrition: Calories 189; Fat 11g; Carbs 35g; Protein 46g

DESSERT RECIPES

Chili's Chocolate Brownie Sundae

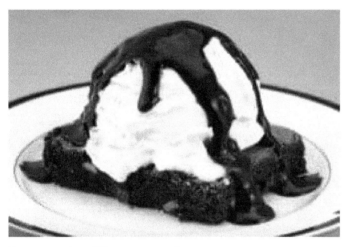

Preparation Time: 20 minutes

Cooking Time: 30 minutes

Servings: 8

Ingredients

- ½ cup flour
- 1/3 cup cocoa
- ¼ teaspoon salt
- ¼ teaspoon baking powder
- ½ cup margarine, melted
- 1 cup white sugar
- 2 eggs

- 1 teaspoon vanilla
- ½ cup chocolate chips
- ½ gallon vanilla ice cream, slightly softened
- 1 (6-ounce) jar fudge topping
- Whipped cream, for topping (optional)
- ½ cup walnuts, coarsely chopped
- 8 maraschino cherries, for garnish

Directions:

1. Preheat oven to 350°F. Grease a 9x9 baking pan. Sift together flour, cocoa, baking powder and salt in a bowl. Set aside.
2. Combine melted margarine, sugar, eggs and vanilla, blending well. Add flour mixture, stirring briefly to moisten. Stir in chocolate chips. Do not over-mix.
3. Pour into prepared pan. Bake until fragrant and corners begin to separate from pan (about 30 minutes). If over-baked, the result will be cakey instead of fudgy.
4. Cool slightly before cutting into 8 bars. Place a scoop of ice cream on top of each brownie and drizzle with fudge sauce. Top with whipped cream (optional) and sprinkle with chopped walnuts.
5. Garnish with cherries.

Nutrition: 1290 Calories 61g Total Fat 14g Protein

Ben & Jerry's Cherry Garcia Ice Cream

Preparation Time: 4 hours

Cooking Time: 0 minute

Servings: 4 - 8

Ingredients

- ¼ cup Bing cherries, fresh or frozen (thawed), drained well and rough chopped
- 2 cups thick cream
- 1 cup milk
- ¾ cup sugar
- 2 large eggs
- 1½ teaspoons vanilla extract (optional)
- ¼ cup semisweet chocolate, broken into bits

Directions:

1. Chill cherries until ready for use. In a saucepan, whisk together cream, milk, sugar and eggs. Whisk while heating gently to 165°F. Remove from heat. Strain into a bowl. Cover and let chill for about 2 hours. Place in ice cream maker and let churn. It should be ready in about 20 minutes. Add cherries and chocolate just before ice cream is done. Transfer to containers, cover, and freeze well (about 4 hours). Serve and enjoy.

Nutrition: 250 Calories 14g Total Fat 4g Protein

P.F. Chang's Coconut Pineapple Ice Cream with Banana Spring Rolls

Preparation Time: 5 minutes

Cooking Time: 30 minutes

Servings: 6

Ingredients

Ice Cream

- 1 (13½-ounce) can coconut milk
- 1 cup granulated sugar
- 1½ cups heavy cream
- 1 teaspoon coconut extract
- 1 (8-ounce) can crushed pineapple, drained
- 1/3 cup shredded coconut

Banana Spring Rolls

- 3 ripe bananas (preferably plantains), halved horizontally
- 3 rice paper or wonton wrappers
- 1–3 tablespoons brown sugar
- 1 teaspoon cinnamon
- Oil, for frying

Caramel sauce, for drizzling (optional)

- Paste for sealing wrappers
- 2 tablespoons water
- 2 teaspoons flour or cornstarch

Directions:

1. Make the ice cream. Place coconut milk and sugar in a mixing bowl. Mix with electric mixer until sugar is dissolved. Mix in remaining ingredients until well-blended. Place in ice cream maker to churn (follow manufacturer's instructions) until ice cream holds when scooped with a spoon (about 30 minutes). Transfer to a container with lid and freeze for at least 2 hours or until desired firmness is reached.

2. Make the banana spring rolls. Lay wrapper on a flat surface. Position a banana slice near the edge of the wrapper closest to you (the bottom). Sprinkle with about 1 teaspoon to 1 tablespoon brown sugar, depending how sweet you want it. Sprinkle with a pinch or two of cinnamon. Roll up like a burrito, tucking in the sides. In a small bowl, stir the paste ingredients together. Brush the paste on the edge of the wrapper and seal the roll. Place roll, sealed side down, on a plate and repeat with the remaining bananas. Heat oil, about 1–1½ inches deep, over medium to high heat. Fry the rolls until golden brown (1–2 minutes on each side). Place on paper towels to drain.

3. Serve the rolls with scoops of ice cream and drizzle with caramel sauce, if desired.

Nutrition: 146 Calories 11g Total Fat 5g Protein

Jack in the Box's Oreo Cookie Shake

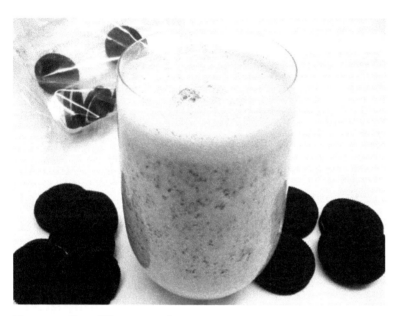

Preparation Time: 5 minutes

Cooking Time: 0 minute

Servings: 2

Ingredients

- 3 cups vanilla ice cream
- 1½ cups milk, cold
- 8 Oreo cookies, without filling, broken into small pieces
- Whipped cream, for topping (optional)
- 2 cherries, for garnish (optional)

Directions:

1. Place ice cream and milk in blender. Pulse gently until smooth. Continue blending at low speed and add Oreos. Blend until cookies are pureed (about 10 seconds). Pour

into 2 cups or glasses. Top with whipped cream and cherries (optional).

Nutrition: 722 Calories 36.4g Total Fat 18.7g Protein

Dairy Queen's Candy Cane Chill

Prep. time: 5 minutes

Cooking time: 0 minute

Servings: 2

Ingredients

- 4 large scoops vanilla ice cream
- 1 cup Cool Whip, thawed or frozen
- ¼ cup milk
- 3 regular sized candy canes, broken into small pieces
- ¼ cup chocolate chunks

Directions:

1. Place all ingredients in a blender. Blend to desired consistency. (Add more ice cream, if needed.) Pour into 2 glasses or mugs.

Nutrition: 536 Calories 26.6g Total Fat 6.6g Protein

Dairy Queen's Blizzard

Preparation Time: 5 minutes

Cooking Time: 0 minute

Serving: 1

Ingredients

- 1 candy bar, of your choice
- ¼ to ½ cup milk
- 2½ cups vanilla ice cream
- 1 teaspoon fudge sauce

Directions:

1. Place the candy bar of your choice into the freezer to harden it. Break the candy bar into multiple tiny chunks and place all the ingredients into a blender.
2. Keep blending until the ice cream becomes thicker and everything is mixed completely.
3. Pour into a cup and consume.

Nutrition: 953 Calories 51.6g Total Fat 15.1g Protein

Houston's Apple Walnut Cobbler

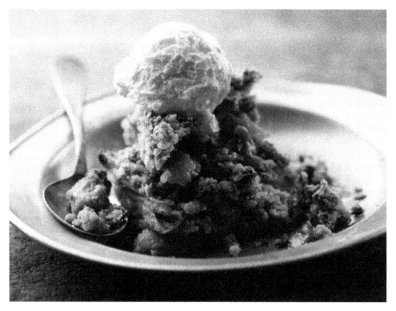

Preparation Time: 15 minutes

Cooking Time: 30 minutes

Servings: 6

Ingredients

- 3 large Granny Smith apples, peeled and diced
- 1½ cups walnuts, coarsely chopped
- 1 cup all-purpose flour
- 1 cup brown sugar
- 1 teaspoon cinnamon
- Pinch of nutmeg (optional)
- 1 large egg
- ½ cup (1 stick) butter, melted
- Vanilla ice cream

- Caramel sauce, for drizzling (optional)

Directions:

1. Preheat oven to 350°F. Lightly grease an 8-inch square baking dish. Spread diced apple over bottom of baking dish. Sprinkle with walnuts.

2. In a bowl, mix together flour, sugar, cinnamon, nutmeg (optional) and egg to make a coarse-textured mixture. Sprinkle over the apple-walnut layer.

3. Pour melted butter over the whole mixture. Bake until fragrant and crumb top is browned (about 30 minutes). Serve warm topped with scoops of vanilla ice cream. Drizzle with caramel sauce (optional).

Nutrition: 611 Calories 36g Total Fat 8g Protein

Melting Pot Chocolate Fondue

Preparation Time: 10 minutes

Cooking Time: 5 minutes

Servings: 4

Ingredients

- 8 ounces semi-sweet or dark chocolate chips
- 1 cup heavy cream
- 1 tablespoon unsalted butter
- 2 tablespoons chunky peanut butter or Nutella (optional)
- Possible complements: strawberry, banana, grapes, cherries, brownies, cream puffs, rice puffs, marshmallows or cheesecake, cut into bite-size pieces

Directions:

1. Heat cream in a saucepan to a simmer. Stir in butter, chocolate, and peanut butter or Nutella (if using). Let sit to allow the chocolate to melt (about 2 minutes). Whisk until smooth and serve immediately with desired complements.

Nutrition: 667 Calories 32g Total Fat 9g Protein

P.F. Chang's Ginger Panna Cotta

Preparation Time: 10 minutes

Cooking Time: 4 hours and 10 minutes

Servings: 3

Ingredients

Panna Cotta:

- ¼ cup heavy cream
- ½ cup granulated sugar
- 1 tablespoon grated ginger
- 1½ tablespoons powdered gelatin
- 6 tablespoons warm water

Strawberry Sauce:

- 2 pounds ripe strawberries, hulled
- ½ cup granulated sugar
- 2 teaspoons cornstarch
- ½ lemon, juice
- 1 pinch salt

Direction:

1. Place the cream, sugar and ginger in a saucepan and cook over medium-low heat, until the sugar dissolves. Remove the mixture from heat and set aside.

2. In a medium-sized bowl, mix the water and the gelatin together. Set aside for a few minutes. After the gelatin has rested, pour the sugar mixture into the medium-sized bowl and stir, removing all lumps.

3. Grease your ramekins and then transfer the mixture into the ramekins, leaving 2 inches of space at the top.

4. Place the ramekins in your refrigerator or freezer to let them set for at least 4 hours.

5. While the panna cottas are setting, make the strawberry sauce by cooking all the sauce ingredients in a medium-sized pan for 10 minutes. Stir the mixture occasionally, then remove from heat.

6. When the panna cottas are ready, flip over the containers onto a plate and allow the gelatin to stand. Drizzle with the strawberry sauce and serve.

Nutrition: 346 Calories 30g Total Fat 4g Protein

MEXICAN RECIPES

Ground Beef Mexican Dip

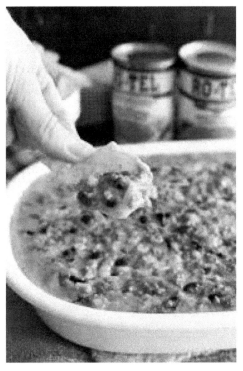

Preparation Time: 25 mins

Cooking Time: 50 mins

Servings: per Recipe: 32

Ingredients:

- 1 lb. ground beef

- mushroom soup
- 1 (16 oz.) jar salsa
- 2 lb. processed cheese food, cubed
- 1 (10.75 oz.) can condensed cream of

Directions:

1. Heat a medium pan on medium-high heat and cook the beef till browned completely.
2. Drain off the grease from the pan.
3. In a slow cooker, transfer the cooked beef with the salsa, condensed cream of mushroom soup and processed cheese food.
4. Set the slow cooker on High till cheese melts completely.
5. Now, set the slow cooker on Low and simmer till serving.

Nutrition: Calories 150 kcal Fat 11.3 g Carbohydrates 3.9g Protein 8.3 g Cholesterol 30 mg Sodium 429 mg

Pepperjack Pizza

Preparation Time: 20 mins

Cooking Time: 32 mins

Servings: per Recipe: 6

Ingredients:

- 1/2 (16 oz.) can spicy fat-free refried beans
- 1 C. salsa, divided
- 1/4 C. crumbled tortilla chips
- 1 (12 inch) pre-baked Italian pizza crust
- 1 C. shredded pepper Jack cheese
- 2 C. shredded hearts of romaine lettuce
- 3 medium green onions, thinly sliced
- 1/4 C. ranch dressing

Directions:

1. Set your oven to 450 degrees F before doing anything else and arrange a rack in the lowest portion of the oven.
2. In a bowl, mix together the beans and 1/2 C. of the salsa.
3. Arrange the crust on a cookie sheet and top with the bean mixture evenly.
4. Cook in the oven for about 10 minutes.
5. Remove from the oven and place the lettuce, green onions over the bean's mixture.
6. Top with the remaining salsa.

7. Drizzle with the dressing evenly and top with the chips and cheese evenly.

8. Cook in the oven for about 2 minutes more.

9. Cut into 6 slices and serve.

Nutrition: Calories 373 kcal Fat 15.3 g Carbohydrates 44g Protein 17 g

Cholesterol 26 mg Sodium 1027 mg

Quick Midweek Mexican Macaroni

Preparation Time: 20 mins

Cooking Time: 50 mins

Servings: per Recipe: 8

Ingredients:

- 1 C. dry macaroni
- 1 (10 oz.) can diced tomatoes with green chili 1 lb. ground beef
- peppers, drained
- 1 small onion, chopped
- 1 (1 lb.) loaf processed cheese, cubed
- 1 (11 oz.) can whole kernel corn, drained

Directions:

1. In large pan of the boiling water, add the macaroni for about 8 minutes.
2. Drain well.
3. Meanwhile, heat a medium skillet on medium-high heat and cook the beef till browned completely.
4. Add the onion and cook till browned.
5. Drain off the grease from the skillet.
6. Reduce the heat to medium and stir in the corn, tomatoes, cheese and cooked noodles.
7. Cook, stirring gently till bubbly.

Nutrition: Calories 374 kcal Fat 21.4 g Carbohydrates 23.5g Protein 22.9 g Cholesterol 79 mg Sodium 997 mg

Cancun Style Caviar

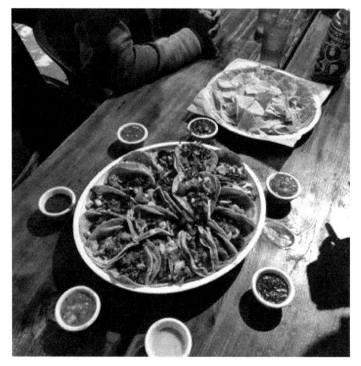

Preparation Time: 10 mins

Cooking Time: 6 h 10 mins

Servings: per Recipe: 32

Ingredients:

- 2 large tomatoes, finely chopped
- 5 green onions, chopped
- 1 (2.25 oz.) can chopped black olives
- 3 tbsp. olive oil
- 1 tsp garlic salt
- 3 1/2 tbsp. tarragon vinegar
- 1 tsp salt

- 1 (4 oz.) can chopped green chili peppers

Directions:

1. In a medium bowl, mix together all the ingredients.
2. Refrigerate, covered for about 6 hours or overnight before serving.

Nutrition: Calories 17 kcal Fat 1.5 g Cholesterol 0.9g Sodium 0.2 g

Carbohydrates 0 mg Protein 188 mg

Puerto Vallarta Eggplant

Preparation Time: 10 mins

Cooking Time: 25 mins

Servings: per Recipe: 4

Ingredients:

- 1 lb. ground beef
- 1 tsp chili powder
- 1/4 C. chopped onion
- 1 eggplant, cut into 1/2-inch slices
- 1 tbsp. all-purpose flour
- salt and ground black pepper to taste
- 1 (8 oz.) can tomato sauce
- 1 C. shredded Cheddar cheese
- 1/4 C. chopped green bell pepper
- 1 tsp dried oregano

Directions:

1. Heat a large skillet on medium-high heat and cook the ground beef and onion for about 5-7 minutes.
2. Drain the grease from the skillet.
3. Sprinkle the flour over the beef mixture and toss to coat.
4. Stir in the tomato sauce, green bell pepper, oregano and chili powder.

5. Sprinkle the eggplant slices with the salt and pepper and place over the beef mixture.

6. Simmer, covered for about 10-15 minutes.

7. Serve with a topping of the Cheddar cheese.

Nutrition: Calories 349 kcal Fat 23.3 g Carbohydrates 6.8g Protein 27.4 g Cholesterol 101 mg Sodium 542 mg

Slow Cooker Nachos

Preparation Time: 20 mins

Cooking Time: 4 h 20 mins

Servings: per Recipe: 15

Ingredients:

- 1 lb. lean ground beef
- 2 -3 cloves garlic, minced
- 1/2 C. chopped green onion
- 2 (16 oz.) packages Velveeta Mexican
- tortilla chips
- cheese, cut into cubes
- 2 (10 oz.) cans Rotel Tomatoes, drained

Directions:

1. Heat a large skillet and cook the beef and garlic until it is browned completely.
2. Drain the fat from the skillet.
3. Transfer the beef mixture in a large slow cooker with the tomatoes and cheese and stir to combine.
4. Set the slow cooker on Low and cook, covered for about 3-4 hours, stirring once after 2 hours.
5. Uncover and stir in the onions.
6. Serve the beef mixture with the tortilla chips.

Nutrition: Calories 241.5 Fat 16.2g Cholesterol 67.4mg Sodium 1067.5mg Carbohydrates 7.6g Protein 16.1g

Licuado de Mango

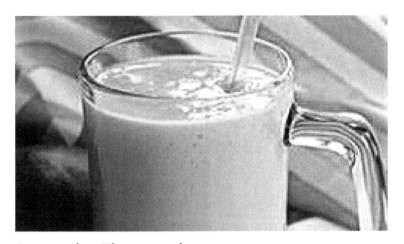

Preparation Time: 10 mins

Cooking Time: 10 mins

Servings: per Recipe: 2

Ingredients:

- 1 mango, peeled, seeded and diced
- 3 tbsps. honey
- 1 1/2 cups milk
- 1 cup ice cubes

Directions:

1. Blend all the ingredients mentioned above until the required smoothness is achieved.
2. Serve

Nutrition: Calories 255 kcal Carbohydrates 52.1 g Cholesterol 15 mg Fat 3.9 g Protein 6.7 g Sodium 82 mg

CONCLUSION

Copycat recipes are the best thing to happen to cooking since the invention of the pressure cooker. I love copycat recipes because they allow me to make something delicious, but in a fraction of the time it takes me to make it from scratch. Copycat recipes are a great way to save money and time. You don't have to rely on specialty ingredients that you may not have access to, or ingredients that you don't know how to use.

Copycat recipes are a great way to make money. It's also an easy way to make some extra cash that doesn't take much effort on your part.

Copycat recipes are a great way of saving time when you're short on time. They can also help to save money because you don't have to buy ingredients in bulk. Copycat recipes are a great way to save time and money. When you get sick of the same old recipes, just make your own! It's not as hard as it sounds. Copycat recipes are great as long as you follow the recipe exactly. That way, you will get a perfect result every time.

Copycat recipes are a great way to save time and money, they are also a good way to learn how to make a recipe. Copycat recipes are awesome because they allow you to create your own personal food experience. You can try new ingredients and experiment with different flavors, and share your results with the world on social media.

If you're going to make a copycat recipe, don't take shortcuts. It's important to follow the recipe exactly and not change the process in any way.

When you're trying to come up with a copycat recipe, you have to think about the original recipe and how it works. You have to pay attention to the flavors used, ingredients used, and ratios. Nazarian has a book called "Copycat Recipes" that offers copycat recipes for over 60 of his favorite dishes from famous restaurants, and it's available on Amazon. Here are the recipes that we've found:

My advice to you is to try some of the recipes in this post. I have tried many of them, and in my opinion they really work well.

There are many copycat recipe sites out there, but not all of them are created equally. Since the book was published, I've seen a lot of copycat recipes for the book. You can find them on Pinterest, Twitter, and see them in more niche blogs as well. Here are some examples: The most important thing when creating a recipe is to make it taste delicious! Your goal should be to make your recipes so good that you don't even need to make a public recipe.

When your recipe is a big hit, don't feel pressured to share it. If you've been asked for a copy and you're not sure how to do so, ask your followers on social media. You may have noticed that I have a copycat recipe on the blog. This post is my best guess at how to make those recipes so you can save time and money.

Copycat recipes are the absolute best! These recipes give you a taste of a brand, without having to pay the full price. They are usually very cheap and can be made in large quantities.

CPSIA information can be obtained
at www.ICGtesting.com
Printed in the USA
BVHW052027120421
604747BV00005B/335